Understand & Manage Diabetes; For Moms, Dads & Kids

After your baby is born it is going to be a relief to not have to take insulin injections anymore or to watch every single thing you put in your mouth. But not so fast, you still need to be careful and mindful of the increased risks that you now face as a mom who has had gestational diabetes…..

There are going to be times when your child is going to need help to manage their diabetes and it may be an emergency situation because their blood sugar has dropped dangerously low. Your child should be wearing identification that advises everyone that they are diabetic and are taking insulin and ……

This complication of Diabetes is not all that well known, by the general Medical Practitioner or the general public, and yet it is extremely debilitating to the sufferer, can be painful in the extreme, and so far as medicine is concerned, incurable….

ISBN-10: 1466350342
ISBN-13: 978-1466350342

i

1. Gestational Diabetes

Gestational Diabetes

According to the American Diabetes Association, about four per cent of pregnant women develop gestational diabetes. Gestational diabetes is a condition in which a woman who has never had diabetes develops high blood glucose levels while pregnant, usually within the later term of the pregnancy. It is estimated that there are about 135,000 cases of gestational diabetes every year in the United States.

In most cases, women who develop gestational diabetes will not develop Type II diabetes. This is a condition affected by the pregnancy and the inability of the mother to use the insulin naturally developed in her body. It is caused by hormones triggered by the pregnancy and causes the mother to become insulin resistant. Gradually, the mother develops high blood glucose levels, referred to as hyperglycaemia.

Normally, a woman with gestational diabetes will be treated for the condition while pregnant. While there are no birth defects associated with this sort of illness as there are with women who have had diabetes prior to being pregnant, there is generally not a large cause for alarm for the child. However, if the condition is left untreated, it can hurt the baby. Because the mother is not getting rid of her excessive blood glucose, the child is getting more than his or her share of energy and fat. This often results in macrosomia. Macrosomia is simply the clinical name for a fat baby.

While some people think a fat baby is the sign of a healthy baby, a child born too fat may have a problem fitting through the birth canal. This can cause shoulder damage and may require a caesarean section birth,. In addition, babies who are born obese can develop breathing problems and, if they remain obese, may themselves develop Type II diabetes.

Fortunately, there is treatment for gestational diabetes. Insulin injections are usually given to the mother to keep the blood glucose levels intact. A woman who is planning on becoming pregnant, however, can avoid the complication of developing gestational diabetes prior to becoming pregnant. Some of the ways a woman can do this is to lose weight if she is already overweight prior to becoming pregnant, develop a healthy exercise routine and follow certain food guidelines. The Glycaemic Index is an ideal tool for a woman who is thinking about becoming pregnant to use to determine which foods to avoid. The Glycaemic Index was developed for diabetics to categorize carbohydrates for those with diabetes.

When you become pregnant, follow the advice from your doctor regarding diet and exercise as well as any carbohydrate diets. Prior to becoming pregnant, discuss any concerns you have regarding weight or diabetes with your physician as he or she can probably give you some advice on how to avoid this pregnancy complication.

Even if you are diagnosed with gestational diabetes, chances are that you will not develop Type II diabetes, neither will your baby and both of you will be just fine. Gestational diabetes is not a reason to panic. There is plenty of care available for women with this condition. Just be sure to follow any instructions given to you by your doctor.

What Is Gestational Diabetes?

When a woman develops insulin resistant during pregnancy it is referred to as gestational diabetes. The disease acts in the same manner as when a person who is not pregnant has diabetes. In most cases, after the baby is born the diabetes goes away and a woman's blood glucose control and insulin production return to normal.

The placenta that provides nourishment and keeps the baby alive as it grows inside the uterus also releases a hormone that effectively blocks or inhibits a woman's insulin production from the pancreas. It can also affect the way a woman's body uses the insulin that is produced. When there is too much sugar (glucose) in a woman's system that is not being converted to energy it produces high blood sugar. This condition is known as hyperglycaemia.

Every woman is routinely screened for gestational diabetes at her monthly doctor's exam during pregnancy. The urine sample that the woman provides is checked for glucose (among other things). If there is glucose in the urine it is a red flag to the doctor to have the woman screened for gestational diabetes. The doctor will then send the patient to a medical lab for blood work and if the results come back positive a referral will be given to an endocrinologist (a doctor specializing in the treatment of diabetics). A treatment and management plan will be put into action for the women to follow for the remainder of the pregnancy.

Although gestational diabetes is a serious condition that affects both the mother and the developing foetus there is no cause for alarm. There are many things known about treating diabetes in pregnancy – although not as much information on why it occurs. With good control of blood sugar levels, following a proper diet, and regular exercise a mom with gestational diabetes can go on to deliver a healthy baby.

What Causes Gestational Diabetes?

The exact cause or causes of what causes gestational diabetes are not known. But there are risk factors that can increase the chances of getting it. As with any disease, risk factors are not a guarantee that you will contract the disease they just make the likelihood of getting it higher. Some of the risk factors you will have control over and some you do not.

A family history of diabetes will increase the chances of developing gestational diabetes in pregnancy. The closer the relative is to you (first generation like a parent) means the risk is increased. If your family suffers from diabetes, your own pancreas may not be able to produce the amount of insulin necessary while pregnant. This deficit combined with the hormones released by the placenta can lead to diabetes in pregnancy.

Women who are overweight and are clinically considered obese run a higher risk of being diagnosed. The excess wait puts a strain on your body, including your pancreas, and makes it hard for enough insulin to be produced and used by your body effectively.

If you have had a previous baby with a higher than average birth weight, you are considered at risk for your next pregnancy of getting gestational diabetes. It could have been possible that you had it in your first pregnancy and it went undiagnosed. Babies born from moms with diabetes in pregnancy tend to be larger unless her blood sugars are strictly managed. Or if you had diabetes in your first pregnancy, chances are very high that you will get it again.

Since there is still no known cause a woman may have all of these factors or none and still get diabetes. It is best to attend all of your prenatal appointments with your doctor so he can be on the lookout for any signs that you may have gestational diabetes.

Treatment Options For Gestational Diabetes

Once you have been diagnosed with gestational diabetes you will see an endocrinologist and develop a treatment plan. You may also see a nutritionist or dietician to help you develop a food plan that will meet the needs of you and the baby and not be detrimental to your blood sugar level.

What you eat will have a major impact on your blood glucose levels. It is not only foods high in sugar that you have to avoid. A good meal plan will make use of the recommended food guide with several small meals spaced throughout the day. Ideally, you should eat six times a day: breakfast, snack, lunch, snack, dinner, and a bedtime snack. By eating frequent and small meals you can keep better control of your glucose level by trying to keep a slow and steady supply of energy for your body. Having a small amount of protein at each meal and snack is beneficial in maintaining a healthy blood glucose level.

Physical exercise is also very important. You can control and lower your glucose levels by getting active. Before you start any physical routine, be sure to consult with your doctor. The exercise you do does not have to be vigorous. You can take three small walks after breakfast, lunch, and dinner for 15-20 minutes to help burn off the extra sugar in your body.

A strict diet and physical exercise are going to be used for any woman with gestational diabetes. But for woman who have higher insulin needs (and the need for insulin is going to increase as the pregnancy progresses) they will have to have additional insulin by way of injections. This isn't as scary as it sounds and it is something you will get used to quite quickly. With the help of your doctor you will learn how to adjust your insulin based on your blood sugar readings from your glucose monitor.

How Is Gestational Diabetes Diagnosed

Each month of your pregnancy you should have a prenatal exam by your health care provider. During your visit to the office or clinic you will provide a urine sample to the nurse. Amongst other things, the doctor or midwife wants to determine if there is in glucose in your urine.

If your body is spilling glucose into your urine, it is a warning sign that you may have gestational diabetes. The next step that your doctor may take is to test your blood sugar level in the office with a glucose monitor. This is a small, transportable device that comes with an electronic reader, lancets, and testing strips. A small pin prick is made on your finger with the lancet and the drop of blood is placed on one of the strips and placed into the reader. Depending on the reading the monitor provides your doctor may or may not order a blood test at the lab.

To be on the cautious side, most doctors will send you for a glucose tolerance test at the lab regardless of the blood sugar level in the office. This is a fasting test and you will not be able to eat for 10 hours before having your blood tested. For this reason, the tests are performed first thing in the morning and you don't eat anything before going to bed.

When you arrive you will have your blood drawn and then be given a drink high in sugar. After drinking this, you will be asked to wait one hour and have your blood tested again. The results of this test will tell how your body is processing the sugar in your body.

If the tests come back positive, most likely you will be referred to a specialist for further care and treatment.

How Exercising Can Help With Gestational Diabetes

Unless you already have a regular fitness routine, you probably don't want to start one half way through your pregnancy. But the benefits that you will derive as a woman with gestational diabetes who exercises will make the physical activity worth it in the end. Before you begin any new physical activity or routine, discuss with your doctor any guidelines you need to follow or warning signs you should heed.

You do need to be aware and careful about when you eat and take your insulin in relation to any physical exercise. If you wait too long after eating to exercise, you will cause your blood sugar to drop dangerously low. A good rule to follow at any time – exercising or not – is to have a snack with you to raise your blood sugar quickly. A good snack is something high in sugar that will raise your blood sugar quickly like a juice box or a piece of fruit. Have a snack with you that is long-acting too, such as a granola bar. You can also purchase glucose tablets for emergencies when you become hypoglycaemic.

The best time to exercise is after one of your main meals. If you can fit in a 15-20 minute walk three times a day it would be ideal. But if you cannot, try and go for a bit of a longer walk at least once per day. When at work go for a walk after lunch or schedule a family walk every night after dinner. If you already have an established exercise routine it is probably safe for you to do more but a vigorous or leisurely walk is extremely beneficial.

Exercising will help you keep your blood glucose levels under control and increase your energy. Getting in shape through exercise before delivery can help your labour progress smoothly as well.

Blood Sugar Guidelines For Gestational Diabetes

In order to diagnose you with gestational diabetes, your healthcare provider will order a test from the lab. There are two levels of the test that can be taken – the one hour glucose tolerance test and the three hour glucose tolerance test.

The one hour test involves taking a blood sample after you have fasted and then drinking a beverage high in glucose and testing your blood again one hour later. With the three hour version, you proceed the same except the drink has a higher concentration of sugar and your blood is tested each hour for three hours instead of one. The purpose of these tests is to see how your body reacts to and process the large amount of sugar in the drinks.

The American Diabetes Association lists the following blood glucose levels that would indicate gestational diabetes is present:

* Fasting 95 mg/dl or higher * One hour 180 mg/dl or higher * Two hours 155 mg/dl or higher * Three hours 140 mg/dl or higher

If any two of the above readings come back in the ranges indicated you will be diagnosed with gestational diabetes. Once you have been diagnosed, you doctor will provide you with the blood glucose guidelines that should be maintained for the optimal health of you and your baby. They are:

* First thing in the morning – below 95 mg/dl * One hour after a meal – below 140 mg/dl * Two hours after a meal – below 120 mg/dl

There will be occasions when your blood sugar reading is higher than the recommended range. In that case, adjust your next meal. If you had planned on having a meal that was higher in carbohydrates it should be changed so that there is more protein. Protein helps to lower your blood sugar and carbohydrates convert to sugar raising your glucose levels.

Gestational Diabetes – Risks For Moms After Pregnancy

After your baby is born it is going to be a relief to not have to take insulin injections anymore or to watch every single thing you put in your mouth.

But not so fast, you still need to be careful and mindful of the increased risks that you now face as a mom who has had gestational diabetes. Even though your health choices do not directly affect your baby as they did when you were pregnant (unless you are nursing), your health is still just as important to take care of for the sake of your baby.

The biggest risk for moms who have had gestational diabetes is a significantly increased chance of contracting type 2 diabetes down the road. It is highly advisable to have a blood screening done six months after the birth of your baby to ensure glucose levels are still being managed properly and that the pancreas is producing enough insulin. After the initial six month screening, an annual test should be conducting to watch for diabetes or a condition known as pre-diabetes.

Women who have had gestational diabetes in a previous pregnancy should consult with their doctor prior to becoming pregnant again. A blood test can be ordered to ensure blood glucose levels are in the normal range which is important in the crucial first weeks of pregnancy.

After giving birth, breastfeeding is the best thing for you and your baby. In addition to the myriad of other benefits that will be derived from breastfeeding it can reduce the chances of your baby developing diabetes later in life.

Taking good care yourself while pregnant can help you reduce the risks associated with diabetes in pregnancy. Continue to eat sensibly and exercise regularly to maintain a healthy body weight – this is crucial to preventing and managing diabetes.

Gestational Diabetes – Risks For Baby

When you first discover that you have gestational diabetes most likely you are going to be upset and worried about your baby. There are risks to the baby when a mother has gestational diabetes but with careful monitoring and strict control of diet and blood glucose levels these risks can be minimized.

The most frequent complication associated with babies whose mothers have had gestational diabetes is how big they become. The extra glucose in the mother's system is also shared by the baby and the baby creates extra insulin which in turn produces unneeded fat stores – this is not healthy for the baby and the baby's size can become dangerous. A large baby (known as macrosomia) can make labour and delivery more difficult. The baby can get injured during delivery (shoulder injuries are common) and a higher percentage of moms with gestational diabetes having a caesarean section.

If your diabetes is poorly controlled while you are pregnant your baby will be born producing more insulin than it should. Once the baby is born and is no longer exposed to your high glucose levels, he or she will still be producing insulin at the same rate they were in the womb. This can cause your baby's own blood sugar level to drop dangerously low, this condition is called hypoglycaemia.

When a baby is born with high insulin levels the effects are long-lasting. The baby will grow up and be at a higher than normal risk of developing type 2 diabetes for the rest of its life. These same babies may also suffer from childhood obesity because of the additional fat stores that were creating during pregnancy. These risks give moms the incentive and drive to stick with the diabetic diet and exercise regime – it is the way to give your baby the best start.

Gestational Diabetes – Risks For Moms During Pregnancy

Even though in most cases gestational diabetes is temporary and is rectified after your baby is born, it is still serious and needs to be managed properly. You will have the support of your doctor and most likely an endocrinologist and a dietician but the actual work of eating properly and exercising falls into your lap. There are risks for your baby if you don't and risks for yourself too.

For moms, the knowledge that having gestational diabetes can cause complications for their unborn child is incentive enough to stick to the diet and exercise even when they are too tired to do so. But, it needs to be done for you too.

One of the complications that is associated with gestational diabetes is high-blood pressure that can lead to preeclampsia in pregnancy – dangerous to both mom and baby. When a baby becomes bigger than average due to mismanaged diabetes during pregnancy, the large size is

13

not good for the mother. It can lead to a more complicated delivery where the baby could be hurt or the mother can have a third or fourth degree tear due to the baby's size. If a baby is considered macrosomic (a term that means obese) it increases the chances that the mother is going to have to have a caesarean section. Having a caesarean section is major surgery and comes with all the risks associated with that including infection.

Having gestational diabetes with one pregnancy significantly increases the chances that you will have it again with subsequent pregnancies. It is wise to be tested for the disease as soon as you fall pregnant to ensure the healthiest pregnancy for both you and your baby. It is best to follow the diabetic diet you were given from your first pregnancy as soon as you know or even before you become pregnant again.

Gestational Diabetes – What Happens After The Baby Is Born

The light at the end of the tunnel with gestational diabetes is that the condition is only present when you are pregnant. In almost all cases once your baby is born your pancreas will continue to produce enough insulin for you and your body will process it properly.

In the rare case where it does not, it is likely that you were diabetic prior to becoming pregnant and the diagnosis did not happen until the routine screening for pregnant women. In either case, your doctor will have you continue to monitor your blood glucose levels after the birth of your baby. At a minimum you should test for two days afterwards but your doctor may request that you test for a period of up to two weeks.

During this time you will not be taking insulin. Your doctor is going to want to see how your body is processing your food without the help of additional insulin. It is recommended to continue with the diabetic diet going forward, it is a healthy way to eat and if you are breastfeeding it will ensure that you and your baby are getting the nutrients you need.

Another reason to continue with the diabetic lifestyle even after it is determined that you no longer have gestational diabetes is to prevent getting type 2 diabetes. You are at an increased risk of becoming insulin resistant (also known as type 2 diabetes) once you have had gestational diabetes. Continue to eat the foods you would have while pregnant and watch your portion sizes. After your doctor gives the okay, resume a routine of physical activity even taking your baby for a walk in the stroller.

You will probably feel a sense of relief once your doctor pronounces you diabetes free and you can concentrate on enjoying your new baby.

The Risk Of Gestational Diabetes In Future Pregnancies

If you are diagnosed with gestational diabetes in pregnancy the chances are very high you will also get the disease in future pregnancies. There have been cases where this hasn't happened and there may be steps you can take to lessen your chances of getting it again.

Before you plan on becoming pregnant again, start to follow the diabetic diet you were given during your previous pregnancy. It will provide a lot of the nutrients your body needs and will start you off on the right track to eating right while pregnant. Maintaining a healthy body weight is also crucial to prevent a reoccurrence of diabetes in pregnancy. If you are overweight, even losing 10-15 pounds before becoming pregnant will help your body better manage the insulin production and use.

A risk factor for getting gestational diabetes in the future is also based on how soon in your pregnancy you were diagnosed. Some woman do not find out they have diabetes in pregnancy until the final weeks before the birth while others may be diagnosed as early as the first trimester. The earlier you are diagnosed the greater the chance that you will also have the same problem again.

When planning your next pregnancy, book an appointment with your doctor. Let him or her know your plans and a blood test will be ordered. Your doctor can order a blood test that will show you average blood glucose levels for the previous few months. This will make sure that before you become pregnant you blood glucose levels are at an optimal level. And if they are not it is recommended that you do not become pregnant until they are under control. Not having your blood sugars under control before you become pregnant can lead to complications for the baby during the crucial first weeks of development.

Preventing Diabetes After Having Gestational Diabetes

After having a taste of what it is like to have diabetes while pregnant you probably want to do what you can to avoid getting type 2 diabetes. The management of diabetes isn't hard but the complications that can occur and having to take insulin daily can take their toll. The good news is there are things that you can do to lessen the chances that you will not be diagnosed with type 2 diabetes.

The same methods that were used during your pregnancy to manage your diabetes can be utilized to help prevent you getting diabetes later in life. Eating a balanced diet is good advice for anyone but for someone that could get diabetes it is even more important. Small meals that include multiple food groups and combining them whenever possible with protein are better choices than large unbalanced meals.

Physical exercise will continue to play a role in your health. It will help your body process the food that you eat and burn off any extra glucose in your system. Activity will give you more energy and if you followed the doctor's orders during pregnancy you should already be in the habit of going for regular walks every day.

If you are overweight, by losing a few pounds you can help your body process the food you consume. In type 2 diabetes you become insulin resistant, your pancreas cannot keep up with your insulin needs and there is a need to supplement with injections or when you are not pregnant you can take an oral pill. But if you lose weight, you will lessen your insulin needs and in turn take the strain off of your pancreas.

These tips may not prevent you from ever getting type 2 diabetes but they will lessen the chances or delay the onset of getting the disease.

When You Get Sick And Have Gestational Diabetes

Aside from the morning sickness that many women suffer from in the first 12 weeks of pregnancy, you may catch a cold or the flu before your baby is born. In of itself, this isn't a fun experience but when you have gestational diabetes and are on insulin it is very important that you take extra good care of yourself.

It is important to remember that no matter how you are feeling, you need to take your insulin. Your body relies on the external source of insulin and needs it to keep functioning properly. But what do you do if you have the flu and are vomiting or don't have any appetite to eat. As a short term solution, take your insulin and drink a soda that is not diet (you want the sugar in this case). If you are able to, nibble on crackers or dry toast. All the while, you need to keep a very close eye on your glucose levels with your monitor.

You need to balance the insulin you are taking and the food you are consuming so your blood sugar levels do not drop. If you are unsure of what to do, contact your doctor. A better plan is to have this discussion with your doctor before you get sick. Your health care provider will give you guidelines to follow when you become ill and when you should contact the office or go to the hospital if things are progressively getting worse.

Getting sick is never fun but being pregnant and sick isn't just about you. You have to still take care of your baby and yourself. Be aware that when you are sick, your blood sugars may not act as they normally do, test more often to keep track of what the results are.

Breakfast Ideas For Women With Gestational Diabetes

Depending on when you are diagnosed with gestational diabetes during your pregnancy (most likely between weeks 24 and 28) you are going to have many weeks of watching what you eat ahead of you. If you find a meal that you like and works well with your blood sugars you may be tempted to eat it again (and again and again).

You are going to reach a point where you do not want to even think about a piece of toast with peanut butter again. And when you do, here are some ideas for a diabetic friendly breakfast:

* One piece of whole wheat toast with 1 tablespoon of natural peanut butter and a glass of milk * A bowl of cereal and milk with almonds sprinkled on top * One egg (cooked to your preference) a piece of toast and a glass of milk * Natural peanut butter spread on half a banana * Egg and cheese omelette with your choice of vegetables

Go for quality foods because as you can see, meal sizes are going to be small. By combining your breakfast foods with a protein you will assist your body in processing the sugar. The added benefit of the protein is be satiating for a longer period of time. If you fill up on carbohydrates (which is very easy to do at breakfast) you are going to be hungry sooner and have a higher blood sugar for your next reading.

As breakfast is going to set the tone for the rest of the day, don't cheat. If you have a high-sugar cereal for breakfast, your blood sugar will be elevated for the rest of the day. After indulging you will have to make up for it during subsequent meals by having less to even out your blood glucose levels.

Lunch Ideas For Women With Gestational Diabetes

A sandwich can be a diabetic's best meal choice. It combines many of the food groups in one easy to prepare meal. Choosing whole wheat bread over white and including a protein increases the nutritious value of the sandwich. But you don't have to be pinned down to eating a sandwich every day for lunch for months on end (unless of course you want to).

Good sandwich choices for diabetics include tuna fish, egg salad, deli meat, and cheese. The addition of vegetables is a good idea and recommended. Be careful with the condiments you add to your sandwich though. Check the labels to get an idea of the sugar content as a guideline mustard is better than mayonnaise and whenever possible go for a lighter or fat free version of your favourite spreads.

If you are looking for ideas that go beyond the four corners of a sandwich try out one of these lunch ideas:

* Instead of making a sandwich with bread try using a tortilla wrap or whole wheat pita pocket * A variety of soups whether homemade or store bought can be hearty and filling. Eat with some cheese slices and crackers for a filling meal * Pasta salad with chicken, ham, or cheese mixed in * Chef's salad with egg and a meat choice. Be aware of how much sugar is in a serving of your salad dressing. A vinaigrette or balsamic vinegar are better choices * A small portion of what you had for dinner the night before

The eating habits you will develop and the food choices that you make when you have gestational diabetes are ones that you would be smart to continue with once the baby is born. Eating like a diabetic is very healthy if you follow the rules and the food guide for portion sizes.

Dinner Ideas For Women With Gestational Diabetes

Dinner is the meal of the day when people like the most variety. You don't want to eat the same thing each night (pregnant or not). Here is the time to be creative. But a cookbook or borrow one from the library to stock up on good ideas for dinner combinations that fit in with your diabetic diet.

The dinner meal traditionally consists of a starch (whole grains, potatoes, and rice), a vegetable, and a protein. You can be creative in how you combine these elements but take the appropriate portions. Your dietician will give you guidelines on is considered a proper portion of meat and other food groups. If you are having difficulty with this, you may want to consider purchasing or borrowing a food scale until you learn how to judge a portion size by sight.

Here is a selection of different dinner ideas that can be made:

* Cheese quiche, you can try making one without the crust to cut fat and calories * Sloppy Joe sandwiches on whole wheat buns topped with shredded cheese (use a lean or extra ground beef) * Bell peppers stuffed with rice and ground beef and then baked in the oven * Use a slow cooker to make a chili or beef stew full of veggies

There are numerous dinner combinations available by mixing up protein choices (fish, steak, pork chops, and chicken) grains (brown rice, potatoes, pasta, and couscous), and the various ways to cook vegetables (raw in a salad, steamed, grilled, or boiled).

If you are going out to eat for dinner, don't be afraid to ask for your food done differently than what the menu offers. Ask for substitutions and sauces on the side where appropriate. Most restaurants are flexible and are willing to accommodate special dietary requirements especially for pregnant women with diabetes.

Restaurant Dining And Gestational Diabetes

It is not expected of you to eat at home for your entire pregnancy but you are going to have to exercise caution when you are dining out in a restaurant or even at a friend's house for that matter. Many foods are not prepared as healthily as they could be but you can make choices and requests that will make eating out less stressful for you and easy on your blood sugar.

Many restaurants today make different eating requirements easy for their clients by designating food choices as "light" or "heart-healthy" these are the ones that should be the first choices on your list. But don't worry; you are not bound to just these choices. Speak up, let your server know of your special dietary requirements and ask if they take special requests or substitutions (very few restaurants will say no).

Here are some ideas of items that can be changed on the menu:

* If you are unsure how a dish is made or with what – ask * Find out how big the meal is. If you know that is a very large portion ask that they box up half before bringing it to you and you will be less tempted to eat more

than you should. * When ordering salad, baked potato, or another item that comes with toppings ask for them on the side if at all.

If you are going to a fast food restaurant it can be even trickier to find something on the menu that is appropriate. But there are some choices available. Steer clear of the fries and look for menu items that include the words broiled or baked. A grilled chicken burger or deli sandwiches are smart choices. Try to stick to your regular eating time, if you arrive at the restaurant early enough you can hope to be served around the same time you would have eaten at home.

Support For Women With Gestational Diabetes

A pregnant woman who has been diagnosed with gestational diabetes is going to receive a lot of medical support in the form of frequent doctor appointments and nutritional counselling. But she may also be in the need of emotional support. It is hard to change the way you eat and live your life when you are pregnant and adjusting to a new disease in addition to that can be overwhelming.

There are many forms of support you can seek out. The support from your spouse or partner is going to be very important. They cannot be eating an ice cream sundae in front of you while you are expected to abstain. Since eating like a diabetic is a healthy lifestyle change, you both should follow the diet set forth for you keeping in mind the extra caloric needs of different people.

Joining a group of pregnant women is helpful too. You can go through your pregnancies together and when your babies are born you can continue with your support network as your children grow up together. Touch base with your endocrinologist to see if they know of a support group specifically for women with gestational diabetes. You can share recipe tips and provide the emotional support needed as you ride the roller coaster of pregnancy with diabetes.

There are many online support groups too with a specialization in many different complications that can arise in pregnancy. Or join a support group for woman online whose babies are due at the same time as yours. You may even meet someone online that lives in your neighbourhood.

Don't feel that you have to deal with your diabetes on your own. Help and support are available. If you can't find it readily with a little research you are sure to find what you need.

2. Type 1 Diabetes

Type 1 Diabetes

Type 1 diabetes accounts for five to ten per cent of diabetes cases in the United States. A person who is diagnosed with type 1 diabetes must receive insulin shots daily in order to live.

Scientists are not exactly sure why the body attacks the immune system and the production of insulin, but it is believed that both genetics and viruses are involved.

Type 1 diabetes is most commonly found in children and young adults, but can appear at any age and symptoms can develop over a short period of time. Symptoms include increased thirst and urination, extreme fatigue, weight loss and constant hunger.

If a person with type 1 diabetes is not diagnosed and treated with insulin, there is a risk of that person slipping into a diabetic coma that may prove life threatening.

The key when first diagnosed with type 1 diabetes is to arm yourself with information. Being diagnosed is not the end of the world. In fact, most people go on to live normal, healthy lives as long as they stay aware of their condition and continue to treat it.

After being diagnosed with diabetes, it is important to maintain your general health paying special attention to the care you give your eyes, feet and skin as well as your heart and oral health.

This basic care could prevent complications brought on by diabetes later in life. Other recommendations are to stop smoking and reduce the amount of alcohol you consume.

What Is Type 1 Diabetes

In type 1 diabetes a person's pancreas is not able to make enough insulin for the body to function properly. Type 1 diabetes is considered an autoimmune disease – the body's cells attack the cells in the pancreas that produces insulin either destroying them entirely or enough of them that there isn't enough insulin.

People who are diagnosed with type 1 diabetes are often surprised because it is not linked to lifestyle or a healthy body weight. As of now, there still is no exact reason that researchers have found that causes a person to develop type 2 diabetes. Although there are risk factors that can increase the chances of someone being diagnosed.

Another name for type 1 diabetes is juvenile diabetes. The reason for this is because the majority of people diagnosed with type 1 diabetes are under the age of 25. There have been reported cases of patients being diagnosed with the disease much older but those are exceptions. There may be a genetic link that causes people to become insulin dependent but the exact link has yet to be discovered.

Diabetics with type 1 will have to take insulin for the rest of their lives. The amount of insulin they take may vary with their diet and weight through the years. Type 1 diabetics need to carefully monitor their urine for ketones every morning as they are more likely to be diagnosed with diabetic ketoacidosis – a serious condition. This is your body's way of telling you it is not getting enough fuel and is using fat cells as energy instead of the food that is being consumed.

The number of people with type 1 diabetes is relatively small compared to the number of people who are being diagnosed with type 2 diabetes. The numbers for type 2 diabetes continue to grow with the obesity rates.

Treatment For Type 1 Diabetes

Type 1 diabetes develops because the cells in the pancreas are not producing enough or any insulin to process the food in the body into energy. The only way to fix this is to inject insulin into the body to replace the insulin the body should be producing on its own. Type 1 diabetes is also known as Insulin Dependent Diabetes Mellitus (IDDM) and requires insulin treatment for the patient to survive. This is done by via insulin injections.

There are two different types of insulin that can be used and in most cases a combination of the two is required. There is fast-acting insulin that is taken and it will start working immediately or within 30 minutes after taking it. This insulin is good for the beginning of the day before breakfast. If your body goes through the insulin quickly another injection of the fast-acting insulin may be required before dinner time. The other type of insulin is long-lasting. It can be mixed with the fast-acting and injected at the same time but can take upwards of 2-3 hours before it takes affect. Taking this insulin the morning should work for lunch or dinner time meals.

If multiple needles to not appeal to you, an insulin pump is another option. It is a machine that will pump fast-acting insulin into your system as needed. Prior to meal times, a button can be pressed to inject an extra dose of insulin to process the food that is going to be eaten. Some find this method offers greater flexibility, a benefit that outweighs the fact the pump has to be worn 24 hours a day.

The other piece of the treatment puzzle is a balanced diabetic diet. In addition to the insulin injections the food that is consumed is very important. If the proper food is not eaten, blood sugar levels will rise and so will insulin requirements.

The Effects Of Smoking With Type 1 Or Type 2 Diabetes

Smoking on its own is associated with many different diseases and can be a risk factor for multiple types of cancer. But in a person with diabetes or a pre-diabetic there are specific risks that arise. There are some differences between type 1 and type 2 diabetes and smoking hazards.

In type 1 diabetes, smoking is not a risk factor for being diagnoses because people with this type of diabetes were born with the genetic make-up to get the disease. But smoking can exacerbate the complications associated with poorly controlled diabetes. An increased risk of heart disease and cardiovascular problems is found in diabetic smokers. In type 1 diabetics who smoke the risk for kidney disease or kidney failure is increased.

In pre-diabetics or people who may be at higher risk to develop type 2 diabetes smoking is a contributing factor to a diagnosis. Smoking increases the likelihood that their body will develop an insulin resistance and need insulin injections or medication in the future.

There are not many studies that have been conducted on the benefits of quitting smoking if you are a diabetic. But it does stand to reason that because smoking and diabetes both increase the chances of heart disease that by quitting smoking you will improve your health and the state of your diabetes.

If you are having trouble quitting on your own or want more information on the benefits of stopping, make an appointment with your doctor. There are many aids that are available as well as support you can utilize to help you in the process. There are nicotine patches and gum or you can try medication or hypnosis. It is a hard thing to do but you will reap many rewards both financially and in terms of your overall health and life expectancy.

Hypoglycaemia And Type 1 And Type 2 Diabetes

Prolonged exposure to high blood sugar levels (hyperglycaemia) will cause long-term damage to your body. But hypoglycaemia, low blood sugars, can cause immediate harmful effects including a diabetic coma. It is important to be able to recognize the signs when your blood sugar is too low and to carry emergency supplies to rectify the situation.

People will react and show different symptoms when their blood glucose levels are too low. They can include some or all of the following:

* Feeling hungry * Feeling nervous or panicked * Feeling light-headed or dizzy * Weakness or lethargy (wanting to go to sleep) * You may be confused, having difficulty speaking or stringing thoughts together. *

Once you have experienced hypoglycaemia a few times you will begin to recognize the signals your body will give you when you need more food in your body. It is important to check your blood sugar with your monitor and have something right away that will act immediately to raise your blood sugars. Hard candies or glucose tablets work fast and are easy to have on you at all times. In case you are not able to help yourself, carry something that identifies you as a diabetic and instructions of what to do and who to call if you need assistance.

Once you have eaten something, test your blood sugar again in 15 minutes to make sure that it is going back to a normal range. You will want to have a snack or a meal too as the burst of sugar will not be long lasting.

By eating small and frequent meals every two to three hours you can lessen the chances of having hyperglycaemia. Another safety precaution that should be taken includes eating prior to exercising and afterwards to keep up your energy level.

Similarities Between Type 1 And Type 2 Diabetes

There are many differences between type 1 and type 2 diabetes – namely how and why a person gets the disease. But there are also similarities. They include how the disease is treated and diabetic diets that are followed.

Once diabetes is diagnosed it is no longer really a matter of why but how to manage it. Whether it is type 1 diabetes and enough insulin is not being produced or it is type 2 diabetes and the insulin that is being produced is not being utilized the solution is to provide more insulin to the body. This is most commonly done with an insulin injection in the morning or spaced out over the course of the day with multiple injections. That will be determined on the individual and their insulin needs – not which type of diabetes they have.

It used to be that type 1 diabetes was found in children or young adults under the age of 25 and type 2 diabetes was diagnosed in adults over the age of 40. There have been many cases to the contrary proving that anyone may be at risk of being diagnosed with type 1 or type 2 diabetes – adults have been diagnosed with type 1 and young children have been found to have type 2 diabetes.

The management of either type of diabetes is also dependent on a healthy diet and regular exercise. By maintaining a healthy body weight and keeping active a person can reduce their insulin requirements and keep their blood sugars in a safe range (set by their doctor).

Despite the different reasons for having diabetes, the two types are very similar in other ways and the treatment plan that works does so for both. Another common trait they share is the complications that can arise to internal organs (especially the kidneys).

The Perception Of Type 1 Diabetes Versus Type 2 Diabetes

It is essentially the same disease in how it affects a person's body but they are completely different in how they develop. In most news and media reports, diabetes is linked with obesity and it is claimed that if more people lost weight or became more active the number of people diagnosed would drop.

These reports can be upsetting to a diabetic with type 1 diabetes, it doesn't matter what their body type is, was, or will be they will always have the disease. There may be some animosity from type 1 diabetics towards type 2 diabetics but this would be misplaced – the media is creating this by not telling the full story.

Yes, type 2 diabetes is intertwined with lifestyle choices and being overweight. This is an epidemic that can be avoided. But not all people diagnosed with type 2 diabetes are considered obese or to be living an unhealthy lifestyle.

Another problem with the misconception about type 1 diabetics is that they make up a very small amount of the people diagnosed with the disease (approximately 10% of all diabetics are type 1). They are not getting as much attention in the news and reports because it is not a growing concern like type 2 diabetes.

It is hard to be diabetic and read the news as it paints type 2 diabetics as people who should just lose weight and they wouldn't have a problem. But it should be noted that there are many people who are overweight and obese who do not have diabetes and the opposite is true too – people who maintain a healthy body weight are being diagnosed with type 2 diabetes.

3. Type 2 Diabetes

Type 2 Diabetes

Type 2 diabetes is the most common form found in the US. Ninety to ninety-five per cent of people diagnosed with diabetes have this type.

Usually developed later in life, it is most commonly diagnosed in people over the age of fifty-five, but in many cases as young as forty or even younger.

This is because eighty per cent of people diagnosed with type 2 diabetes are overweight. With obesity at an all-time high, the diagnoses for type 2 diabetes is also at an all-time high.

In type 2 diabetes, the pancreas is still producing insulin, but for some unknown reason, the body is not able to utilize it effectively. As a result, just as in type 1 diabetes, type 2 people develop a dangerous build-up of glucose in the blood and the body is not able to utilize it for fuel.

People who have type 2 diabetes may see their symptoms develop over time. They are not usually as noticeable as the type 1 symptoms.

Symptoms include fatigue, frequent urination, especially throughout the night hours, unusual thirst, weight loss, frequent infections and slow healing sores.

In fact, sores may never heal and if not treated it is common for people to have limbs amputated. This usually occurs in the legs, feet and toes.

Also as with type 1, if the symptoms go untreated and insulin is not administered when necessary, the patient runs the risk of slipping into a diabetic coma, which can be fatal.

It is important if you have any symptoms of type 1 or 2 diabetes you speak with a health professional and get tested.

What Is Type 2 Diabetes

Where type 1 diabetics do not produce enough insulin for their body, type 2 diabetics produce the insulin but their bodies are not make proper use of it. Type 2 diabetes has been linked to lifestyle choices as a large number of people who are diagnosed are considered overweight or obese. The extra weight a person carries around can make it hard for the body to process insulin properly.

Some additional risk factors for being diagnosed with type 2 diabetes include a family connections (a first or second generation family member) and race. Even with these risk factors present a person can prevent out put-off a diagnosis off type 2 diabetes by losing weight, eating a healthy diet, and plenty of physical activity.

Type 2 diabetes has in the past been diagnosed in patients over the age of 40 but in recent years people of all ages have been diagnosed with this disease. There is an alarming number of young children who are being diagnosed with type 2 diabetes who are obese.

People who have not yet been diagnosed with type 2 diabetes may exhibit some of these symptoms: Urinary Tract Infections (UTI) and skin infections. Moodiness and irritability may also be a symptom of diabetes but is usually not one that precipitates a trip to the doctor and is later explained by high or low blood sugar levels. Other warning signs for type 2 diabetes are the same as type 1 diabetes such as an increased need to urinate, a desire to drink more and a feel of lethargy or constant tiredness.

Type 2 diabetics have a range of options for treatment depending on personal preference and their individual needs in contrast to type 1 diabetics whose only option is to go on insulin injections or an insulin pump.

Treatment For Type 2 Diabetes

In type 2 diabetes, the body is still producing insulin but it is not being utilized properly. This is known as insulin resistance. When a person is diagnosed with type 2 diabetes, there are more treatment options available to them as opposed to people diagnosed with type 1 diabetes.

Depending on the blood sugar levels in a patient, their weight and other health factors, the doctor will decide whether the diabetes can be controlled by one of the following methods:

* Diet and exercise – a healthy balanced diet with regular exercise can be used for people newly diagnosed with type 2 diabetes whose blood sugar levels are only slightly elevated * Oral medication – is for patients whose blood sugars are higher than they should be but not to the point that necessitates an injection of insulin * Insulin injections – a daily injection (or more) of insulin is needed when higher blood sugars are present

A type 2 diabetic may cycle through the different treatment methods throughout their lifetime. It is based on how well they are managing their diabetes and how their body is reacting to the treatment plan. Some people will never have to go past the diet and exercise portion and can gain control by maintaining a healthy body weight and eating the right foods on a diabetic diet.

Other people may start at diet and exercise but as the disease progresses may have to move from oral medication to injections over time. These changes will be determined by your doctor based on physical check-ups and the results of your daily blood sugar monitoring. If you would like to cut back on your medication or the type of treatment you are on, speak to your doctor about your goal and a plan can be put in place to better manage your diabetes.

Complications In Type 1 And Type 2 Diabetes

The long-term effects of improperly managed diabetes on your body and internal organs can be very serious. The different complications range from eye to heart problems and in severe cases can cause premature death.

Heart disease is the leading cause of deaths in diabetics. The best way to prevent damage to your heart is to follow your diabetic meal plan and participate in some form of physical activity every day. By quitting smoking you can decrease the chances of developing any heart problems later on in life. Eating a diet low in saturated fats will promote good heart health and a normal blood pressure too.

If blood sugar levels are not controlled they can lead to serious eye and sight problems including blindness. High glucose in your systems will make small veins in your eyes start to bleed. A regular check-up with an ophthalmologist to check for any signs of damage is recommended once per year. To prevent this, keep your blood sugars under control.

Kidney failure is most common in diabetics who do not control their blood sugars for extended periods of time. When the kidneys fail they are no longer able to clean the blood. After kidney failure the only two options for treatment are dialysis (you are hooked up to a machine that cleans your blood) or a kidney transplant.

Diabetics should take extra care of their gums and teeth as they are more susceptible to gingivitis and other gum disease. A semi-annual check up at the dentist with a regular brushing and flossing routine will help to prevent this disease and the potential loss of your teeth.

All of these complications can be avoided or lessened by the proper management of your diabetes. By following the guidelines set for you by your doctor and checking your blood sugars daily you can lead a long and healthy life with diabetes.

The Difference Between Type 1 And Type 2 Diabetes

To an outsider, the difference between type 1 and type 2 diabetes may be confusing. They are both similar disease that require insulin in order to manage the diabetes and have a properly functioning body. But where it gets confusing is the reason why the two different types of diabetics need the insulin and which one has different treatment options.

Type 1 diabetes is not about lifestyle choices or a person's weight; when a person is born their genetic make-up already make it likely they are going to be diagnosed with type 1 diabetes. In most cases the diabetes is diagnosed in childhood and that is why it is referred to as juvenile diabetes. Type 1 diabetics will have a choice of daily insulin injections (sometimes more) or an insulin pump that provides a steady supply of insulin to the body. An insulin pump also has the ability to provide a bolus (extra insulin) before meal times or when needed. Type 1 diabetes can be managed by the options available for treatment is limited.

Type 2 diabetes is linked to obesity and hereditary factors. In the majority of people who are diagnosed they have a close family member who has diabetes (a parent, grandparent, or a sibling) and they are typically overweight or obese. There are choices available to people with type 2 diabetes in how it is treated. It can be controlled by diet, oral medication, or insulin injections. The choice will be made with the help of your doctor and the severity of your disease. If you get your diabetes under control it is entirely possible that you can downgrade your treatment method (from insulin injections to oral medication).

Diabetic Peripheral Neuropathy

This complication of Diabetes is not all that well known, by the general Medical Practitioner or the general public, and yet it is extremely debilitating to the sufferer, can be painful in the extreme, and so far as medicine is concerned, incurable.

Type 2 Diabetics are particularly at risk of Peripheral Neuropathy if they have not been really aware of their blood glucose levels, and have allowed it to reach even slightly unacceptable levels for a prolonged length of time.

Nerves are enclosed in a myelin sheath, and it is this sheath that is damaged, thereby exposing the nerve ends, and causing pain that has been described as "A Thousand Bee Stings". I speak from experience, and that description is no exaggeration.

The trouble shows as a numbness of feeling in the extremities, usually the feet at first. The numbness becomes a tingling, then progresses to feeling like a bad case of sunburn, on the soles of the feet, or palms of the hands.

These effects are particularly noticeable at bedtime, and the irritation makes sleep almost impossible.

But there is more!

The irritation then degenerates into a jagged pain, which is unpredictable, randomly spread over the affected areas, and so intense that it can extract an involuntary yelp from even the toughest of men/women.

I wish that, when I first became aware of the feeling of numbness in my toes, I had known about Neuropathy being such a serious complication of Diabetes, because I most certainly would've been on my guard, and taken precautions against it.

The numbness continued for a couple of years, but although I wondered about it, I wasn't unduly concerned. I was aware of my diabetes, and was on the maximum amount of medication, also observing dietary restrictions, and was leading a very active lifestyle. I felt that everything was under control.

But then I had to retire to a less active life, and exercising became very difficult due to a couple of very painful knees. I suppose that had I known about Neuropathy and Diabetes at that time, I might have been a lot more particular about my diet. My blood sugar levels always checked out OK, but then the numbness became a tingling, the tingling turned into a burning sensation, then very quickly the full on pain started.

It was at this time that I was told that I had developed Diabetic Peripheral Sensory Neuropathy.

If only I had known that this was coming, a couple of years before!

I was put on Lyrica, an anti-epilepsy drug, and it certainly helped to reduce the pain back to the tingling sensation, but at a price.

Lyrica is not available on our Australian Pharmaceutical Benefits Scheme, and was costing me $AU 200 per month, but the real price was the Zombie-like state that I lived in.

I now do not use Lyrica, but have increased my dose of Effexor, a SNRI antidepressant, and when the pain comes back I hook myself up to a TENS unit for an hour or so. And it does help.

So, be aware, if you've got Type 2 Diabetes, and numb toes, you can probably stop the Neuropathy from becoming worse.

Treatment of Peripheral Neuropathy

Diabetic sensory neuropathy, or nerve pain, triggered by long term diabetes, can be acute, non-stop, and challenging to deal with. It usually begins as a tingling feeling in the feet or hands, then a numbness, and eventually, pain. However, if you do have diabetic peripheral neuropathy, you should remember two important facts:

- You are able to improve your general health, and stop the nerve pain from becoming worse just by controlling your blood sugar levels.

- New medications are being developed all the time that can assist in easing nerve pain, improve your comfort, and enhance your living.

It is a confirmed fact that by controlling blood sugar, neuropathy can be prevented, but if you already have it, its progress can be slowed, and some of the symptoms eased.

Should you have diabetes as well as diabetic neuropathy, discuss alternative methods of blood sugar control with your doctor. It may be necessary for you to take insulin.

After you've got, and can keep, your blood sugar levels at a safe level, including medication, exercise, diet and meal planning; your doctor will be able to assist in choosing the best pain relieving medication for your remaining symptoms.

The ever increasing range of drugs suitable for easing the symptoms of diabetic sensory neuropathy, can permit you to enjoy a near-normal work life. The list of pain easing medicines is long. Several different drugs may have to be tried before one is found that actually assists you.

Non-prescription relief of diabetic nerve pain.

Certain people find relief for slight diabetic nerve pain right on their drug store shelves. Some common analgesic creams and/or pills could possibly help with some of the very minor instances of pain.
As an initial line of treatment, such medicines can be very useful, on the other hand, someone with diabetes ought speak to their doctor prior to taking any other medication. Even over-the-counter remedies can react with other drugs or result in extreme side effects in people with diabetes

A few off-the-shelf pain easing medications .

NSAIDs (non-steroidal anti-inflammatory drugs). These medications reduce inflammation and soothe pain. NSAIDs that may be used are aspirin, naxopren, and ibuprofen, and no prescription required.
But NSAIDs can trigger damaging side effects such as stomach irritation and haemorrhaging in a few people if taken for many weeks. If used over a lengthy period, NSAIDs can cause liver and kidney damage, which is highly likely in diabetics.
However, in many cases, particularly with younger individuals who are reasonably healthy, the danger is rather low.

- Acetaminophen. Acetaminophen and other off-the-shelf medications that contain acetaminophen can ease the diabetic nerve pain, but do nothing to reduce inflammation. These medicines are not as savage on the stomach as NSAIDs are. Make sure that you observe all the directions regarding dosage of acetaminophen, and if in doubt, check with your pharmacist, because liver damage could result if the specified dosage was exceeded.

- Capsaicin. A substance that occurs naturally in chili peppers, Capsaicin is marketed under different brand names such as Capzasin-P and Zostrix. Capsaicin has demonstrated its ability to soothe pain, but there is some worry. It may not be the ideal method. Capsaicin is believed to relieve pain by lowering the quantity of a compound called Substance P, which is active in transmitting pain impulses through the nerves.
Although this may be an effective approach over the short-term, the long-term effects are worrying. These are the nerves that are important in wound healing. We're worried that Capsaicin could deter that recovery, which is already a big problem for diabetes patients.

- Lidocaine is an anaesthetic which de-sensitizes the area it has been applied to. Marketed as Xylocaine or Topicaine, it's available both off-the-shelf and by prescription as a gel or cream.

- More topical creams or gels.

- Salicylate is a compound equivalent to aspirin, and is identified in pain-relieving ointments such as Bengay and Aspercreme.

- Cortisone products consist of corticosteroids, and are effective anti-inflammatory medicines that can help soothe pain.
Both of these preparations are available over-the-counter, but whether they help to ease nerve pain caused by peripheral neuropathy has not been confirmed.

Prescription Drugs for Diabetes Nerve Pain

Should you require a doctor's script for diabetes nerve pain relief, your choices include:

- NSAIDs. Although some drugs are obtainable over-the-counter, your physician may recommend a higher dose, or a different NSAID, that need a script. Although there are plenty of script only NSAIDs available, diabetics are particularly susceptible to kidney damage that can result from prolonged use of NSAIDs. Besides, these script only NSAIDs could increase the risk of heart disease, particularly in diabetics who already have a big chance of developing that problem.

- Antidepressants. Whereas originally, antidepressants were produced for depression, they have also come to be beneficial in relieving extreme pain, whether or not the person is depressed. These drugs have been prescribed by doctors for the control of pain for several years, and include TCAs (Tricyclic Anti-Depressants) mainly affect the levels of norepinephrine and serotonin in the brain. These TCAs have been extensively studied, are the most utilized, and are the most beneficial of the anti-depressants which are used for pain relief.

Tricyclic Antidepressants (TCAs)

Elavil is a good option for pain relief, but has some worrying side effects. Drowsiness, weight gain, dry mouth and eyes. Also, for sufferers of peripheral neuropathy, it has added problems of blood pressure, heart rate, and dizziness.

Pamelor is effective, with fewer side effects, and is better tolerated.

Norpramin. Is also good and has the least side effects of all.

The Newer Antidepressants.

Selective serotonin reuptake inhibitors (SSRIs).
SSRIs are relatively a new antidepressant, and work by changing the amount of serotonin in the brain. Effective for depression, but less so for pain.

Serotonin and norepinephrine reuptake inhibitors (SNRIs).
SNRIs treat depression by increasing accessibility of the brain compounds serotonin and norepinephrine. Effexor and Cymbalta are very effective for pain. They are both as effective as SSRIs or TCAs, but have fewer side effects.

Also

Anti-seizure drugs.
Drugs that were originally developed to prevent epileptic seizures can relieve neuropathic pain. They work by managing the abnormal firing of nerve cells - in the brain and in other parts of the body, like legs and arms.

Neurontin is the anti-seizure drug most frequently chosen for nerve pain from peripheral neuropathy. It can cause sedation or dizziness at larger dosages, but if the dose is raised slowly, it is quite easily tolerated. Lyrica is an anti-seizure drug that is approved for peripheral neuropathy pain by the US FDA, but not by the Australian PBS. The most common side effects are giddiness and sleepiness.

And

Opioid Drugs.
Opioids such as Ultram or Ultracet are used conjointly with Neurontin, which gives immediate relief from pain, and allows the dosage of Neurontin to be slowly increased.
Ultram and Ultracet are painkillers that contain Tramadol, and they also have an effect on the brain chemicals, which reduces the awareness of pain.
Doctors specializing in neuropathic pain prefer not to use strong Opioids due to the common resistance of patients towards using narcotic drugs. There could also be a problem, depending on the sort of work that the patient does.

Additional Therapy Options for Nerve Pain.

- Injections of local anaesthetics such as lidocaine - or patches containing lidocaine.

- Surgically destroy nerves or relieve a nerve compression that causes pain.

- Implant a device that relieves pain.

- Perform Transcutaneous Electrical Nerve Stimulation using a TENS unit which may relieve pain.

And What Of The Future?

A new line of attack on Diabetic Peripheral Neuropathy related pain could be in view, with the development of Metanx. But I need to do a lot more research on this.

4. Diabetes in Kids

Diabetes In Children

Diabetes in children is also known as juvenile diabetes, but more commonly known as type 1 diabetes. It is the most common form of diabetes in children with ninety to ninety-five per cent of carriers being under 16.

Juvenile diabetes is caused by the inability of the pancreas to produce insulin. It is an autoimmune disease, which means the body's own defence system attacks the body's tissues or organs.

In the last 30 years the number of juvenile diabetes had increased three times over and in Europe and the US we are now seeing type 2 diabetes in children for the first time.

Obesity easily explains type 2, but not why there is such a rise in type 1 diabetes in children. It is believed that a mixture of genetics and environmental factors are what triggers juvenile diabetes. But the majority of children don't have a family history of diabetes.

The symptoms for juvenile diabetes are the same as in adults. Thirst, weight loss, fatigue, frequent urination is typical, but diabetes in children can also increase stomach pains, headaches and behaviour problems.

Doctors should consider the possibility of diabetes in children who have unexplained stomach pains for a few weeks, along with the typical symptoms.

If you believe your child may be experiencing these symptoms you should schedule them for a thorough examination and tell your doctor what you suspect your child may have. Be sure to tell them about any and all symptoms your child may be experiencing.

What Is Juvenile Diabetes?

Juvenile diabetes is the onset of type 1 diabetes mellitus in children. Very much the same as the disease in adults, when a child has diabetes their bodies are unable to make enough insulin or they cannot make proper use of the insulin that is made. When a child has type 1 diabetes, daily insulin injections are necessary for the rest of their lives.

Children are diagnosed with juvenile diabetes when their pancreas (the organ that produces insulin) does not make enough insulin on its own or not enough to process the food that is eaten into glucose. Glucose is how our bodies get energy from the food we eat. If a child's body is not processing the food the sugar (glucose) is spilled into the urine without being used for energy. Juvenile diabetes is also known as an autoimmune disease. The child's cells destroy the cells in the pancreas that are needed to make insulin.

There are greater risks and complications associated with diabetes when it exists in young children. A good health care team and due diligence on the parents" part is going to be needed to ensure the child receives the best care possible. As a parent you will have to check your child's blood sugar levels regularly using a blood glucose monitor. It will also be your responsibility to ensure that a proper diet and regular physical activity are part of your child's life.

It is important that other people who care for your child when you are not around know that he or she has diabetes. They need to know what to do in case of an emergency and the special dietary requirements your child requires. It is recommended to get a bracelet or other form of identification that your child can wear that advises they have juvenile diabetes.

The Symptoms Of Juvenile Diabetes

If diabetes runs in your family, you may already be aware of the symptoms to look for to see if your child might have juvenile diabetes. If the disease is prevalent in your family, your doctor may run routine screening tests as a precautionary measure in the form of blood work. But this isn't always the case. If your child exhibits any of the symptoms listed below you should schedule an appointment with your health care provider to have them looked into.

If your child is exhibiting these symptoms, they could be a sign that he or she has juvenile diabetes:

* Extreme thirst – this can be defined as a need to drink constantly without be satiated. * Going to the bathroom to urinate more than usual. In some cases your child may wet the bed because of the increased need to urinate. * Vision difficulties. Your child is complaining that they cannot see things properly or that they are blurry. * Losing weight, you may notice a sudden drop in your child's weight that is not linked to any other causes such as a recent bout of the flu. * Mood changes, the highs and lows of your child's blood sugar can cause them to be grumpy or bad-tempered with little provocation. * A constant desire to eat, this is considered a symptom when the amount of food your child wants to eat is more than normal. * Suffering from stomach aches or pangs with our without vomiting.

All of the above symptoms could mean that your child has diabetes but only blood work ordered by your doctor will prove that. Another point to note is that the above symptoms do not develop over time; it may be quite obvious to you that something is amiss as these changes can happen quite abruptly.

When Diabetes Attacks Kids

Contrary to popular belief the only older people suffer from chronic diseases such as diabetes, more and more kids are now are diagnosed with this illness all over the world. The type of diabetes that kids are prone with is the 'type 1 diabetes." Also known as " juvenile diabetes," this type is diagnosed in almost 40 children every day in the United States of America alone.

Type 1 diabetes can be considered as the rarest type compared to other diabetes types such as 'type 2 diabetes" and "gestational diabetes" but now, more and more people—especially the younger ones suffer from it. Type 1 diabetes usually occurs person's body is stopped form producing enough insulin, which is a type of hormone that every human needs. In order to survive, people—especially kids—with this type of diabetes should have insulin injected in their bodies every single day in order to continue living.

With the help of modern technology, kids with type 1 diabetes can live a normal life because they have better options in terms of blood glucose testing and insulin administration which are just some of the common processes that diabetics undergo. To help kids cope with their condition, more and more medical facilities now offer treatments that can help the child live an active, healthy, and a life filled with fun excitement just like other regular kids.

Dealing with diabetes in children

Parenting a child is enough challenge for a parent once he or she has decided to form a family. But when a child is diagnosed with a chronic illness such as diabetes, parenting and raising this child become more difficult, challenging and at times, frustrating. To help parents deal with their children when diabetes attacks them at such an early age, experts say that they should:

1. encourage and help the child to develop healthy eating habits. Once a child is diagnosed with diabetes, it makes his or her world smaller. There will be more restrictions especially in eating. These restrictions can lead to eating problems that will be harder to manage once they get older. So as early as now, parents must instil among their kids the importance of eating healthy and well-balanced food to avoid further diabetes complications. Parents must also make sure that the child follows the regular schedule in taking in snacks and eating meals. But if the child doesn't want to eat a certain type of food you're offering, don't force him or her. Instead, give the child a variety of healthy foods that he or she can choose from.

2. ensure to test blood glucose levels regularly. The ideal frequency of blood glucose testing is at least four times per day. If possible, the parents should monitor this themselves to ensure that if the child is coping up with the condition or not.

3. instil in the child the importance of regular exercise. To avoid being obese that can lead to more complications among kids with diabetes, parents must make exercise a part of the child's daily living. This exercise should not be so rigorous, it can be a simple walk, jog, or even helping out with household chores as long as there's enough movement for the day.

4. reassure the child of your love and support. There are kids with diabetes who think that having the chronic illness is their fault. Many of them also think that they have that condition because they did something bad or they

are not just good enough for their parents. To erase these doubts in the child's mind, parents must always ensure their child that they will support him or her no matter and they will love the child no matter what.

Childhood Obesity And Type 2 Diabetes

When a child is diagnosed with diabetes it is commonly referred to as juvenile diabetes or type 1 diabetes. This type of diabetes is not related to a child's lifestyle, it is an autoimmune disease that results in the need for insulin injections for food to be turned into energy properly. In recent years there have been an increased number of children that have been diagnosed with type 2 diabetes. This is an alarming trend and one that can be mitigated because the link between children and type 2 diabetes is childhood obesity.

As it is fairly new that children are being diagnosed with type 2 diabetes there isn't a lot of information or studies on it presently. But what is known is that parents need to take action immediately. Once a child has been diagnosed at an older age there isn't much that can be done except to manage the disease. But if a younger child is obese and makes healthy lifestyle changes that result in weight loss there is a chance that type 2 diabetes can be avoided.

Some of the early warning signs that your child may have diabetes include:

* A sudden increase in thirst that appears to never be satiated * An increased need to urinate * Dark patches on the skin – usually found in the folds of the skin, around the neck or around the eyes

As there are many other diseases and complications that can arise if your child is obese it is best to seek medical help for your child. Between you and your health care professional, a plan can be made and put into place that will start your child on the road to a healthier weight and more active lifestyle. Your child may be resistant at first but by involving them in the process and persistence the changes can be made.

How Juvenile Diabetes Is Diagnosed

It can be scary when you realize that something may be wrong with your child. You will want to find out right away what it is and how you can help. The testing that is done to determine if your child has juvenile diabetes is not very evasive and can be determined in a very short period of time.

Once you have taken your child to your health care provider, blood work will be ordered to check your child's blood glucose levels. The first test that is performed is normally a with a blood glucose monitor in your doctor's office. If the level is high a fasting blood glucose test will be ordered. Your child will not be able to eat for 8-10 hours prior to the blood being drawn. It is best to do this first thing in the morning as soon as your child wakes up. Bring a snack along for your child to eat after the blood work as they are sure to be hungry.

Depending on the results from the fasting blood test your doctor will probably order another round of tests to verify the results. This test is also done on an empty stomach and you should make an appointment as you will have to be in the office from 1-3 hours. When you arrive at the lab your child will have some blood drawn and then be asked to drink a beverage that is high in sugar. After one hour another blood test will be conducted to see how your child's body has processed the sugar. If the three hour test was ordered, two more blood tests will be done at the two hour and three hour marks.

The results from this test will give your doctor the information needed to make a diagnosis of juvenile diabetes in your child.

Checking For Ketones In Juvenile Diabetics

Another part of the routine for monitoring and controlling juvenile diabetes is checking for the presence of ketones. This is done by dipping a stick available at drug stores into your child's urine. If ketones are present the end of the stick will turn a certain colour. By matching the colour of the stick with the legend on the container you can determine the level of ketones present.

You should check for ketones first thing in the morning before your child eats (fasting). Give your child additional insulin and fluids if there are ketones present. Also, check again in a few hours and if the test is still positive you should check with your doctor for further instructions.

When there are ketones in urine it is a sign that your child's body is not getting enough food and it is using fat stores for energy instead of food. Excessive ketones can lead to a condition known as ketoacidosis. This is a very serious condition and can even be life threatening. In addition to the presence of ketones you child may be very tired, have trouble breathing, and have stomach pains or nausea.

Ketoacidosis will be present if your child's body does not have enough insulin to process the food he or she is eating or if they are not eating enough. The good thing about this condition is that it is easy to prevent with careful monitoring and by following a meal plan. If you discover ketones, it does not mean that your child has ketoacidosis. Increase the amount of insulin that is being given in addition to reviewing recent diet changes to try and rule out the reason for the ketones.

As in all cases when you have questions about juvenile diabetes, contact your health care provider or diabetes educator.

Having Juvenile Diabetes And Going To School

The vital step after your child is diagnosed with juvenile diabetes is to develop a support network in the community. Your child's school should be at the top of this as a resource to tap into. Not only is it essential that the teachers at your child's school know about his special dietary needs and what to do in an emergency they can provide help in other ways too.

In addition to good control of blood glucose levels to ensure the current and future well- being of your child's health, good control of diabetes is critical to learning. When a child is experiencing highs or lows in the blood sugar reading this can create disruptions and make it hard for them to concentrate and learn.

The teachers or other support personnel are going to need instruction for handling your child's diabetes and what to do in case of an emergency. For a child with a low blood sugar it is important that their blood glucose level is checked and that they have something to eat. For a child with a high blood sugar, their blood glucose will need to be checked too and a decision has to be made whether or not to give insulin. This is a big responsibility to hand over to another adult and can be nerve-racking for parents.

An emergency kit should be with your child at all the time with instructions on what to do to help if something is wrong. Included should be a snack, a food item or glucose tablet that is fast acting (gets sugar into the system quickly), a list of emergency numbers to call, and a glucose monitor. A teacher or school nurse should be designated as the person responsible for your child while at school and they should have a back-up in case they are not present for a day or more.

Complications Associated With Juvenile Diabetes

As with any disease there are possible complications and side effects and juvenile diabetes is no exception. The risks and complications associated with this disease are serious but can be mitigated with careful monitoring and control of your child's blood sugars.

All people that have been diagnosed with diabetes need to have their eyes checked on a regular basis. It is common to have eye problems that are known as diabetic retinopathy. This is when the blood vessels in the eyes are damaged because of raised continually raised blood sugars.

Another complication is diabetic nephropathy. This is a problem that develops in the kidneys taking the form of degeneration or a complete shut-down. This is a very serious disease and should be kept in mind as an important reason to keep blood glucose levels under control at all times. If diabetic nephropathy does develop, it will usually occur later in adulthood but will require either dialysis or a transplant.

Some more long-term effects children with diabetes are exposed to are heart disease, strokes, and hypoglycaemia. But the severity of the complications and the likelihood of them occurring are dependent on how well the diabetes is controlled.

Research continues everyday on ways to better treat and manage diabetes in children. As soon as your children are old enough to understand the disease, involve them in the management of keeping it under control. They need to learn what is needed of them when they become independent to live with diabetes and lessening the chances of suffering from severe complications.

There have been big strides in the treatment of diabetes which has made it possible to delay our put off altogether some of the more troublesome problems. If you suspect that any of the above mentioned diseases are developing, consult with your doctor right away. Early detection is beneficial.

A Juvenile Diabetic's Emergency Kit

An emergency or first aid kit can be found in almost any home. But in a home where a child lives with juvenile diabetes there needs to be additional supplies for their needs. In addition to an at-home emergency kit, a child with diabetes should carry a portable kit with supplies with them at all times.

There are going to be times when your child is going to need help to manage their diabetes and it may be an emergency situation because their blood sugar has dropped dangerously low. Your child should be wearing identification that advises everyone that they are diabetic and are taking insulin and a kit with the supplies needed to help them.

The kit should include instructions on what to do in case of an emergency and numbers to call (parents and health care providers). In addition glucose tablets, fast-acting food stuff should be included to raise your child's blood sugar quickly. Good examples of these are juice boxes and hard candies. You should include a snack that is considered long-acting too. Something that will keep for a long time such as a granola bar is a convenient item to have. This is for situations where your child should be eating their next meal but unavoidably does not have access to food (in the car during a traffic jam or out with friends).

For your home emergency kit, you should include a means to keep your child's insulin cold in the case of a prolonged power outage. A small cooler will work nicely for this. It is also a good idea to always have extra insulin on hand. Do not wait until you are out to pick up more, you never know when an emergency can happen that would prevent you from getting some – be prepared.

Healthy Eating Guidelines For Juvenile Diabetes

A daily insulin injection is required to manage type 1 diabetes in children but it is not the only management strategy. The diet plan that goes along with the daily insulin requirements is just as important and needs to be planned accordingly. Consistency in meal times, portion sizes, and food groups are the keys to successful meal planning for children with diabetes.

Even though consistency is of the utmost importance, it does not mean that your child cannot have variety too. This may seem impossible but there are ways it can be achieved. The important rules to remember are feeding your child at the same time each day and giving them their insulin injection(s) at the same time too. This helps their bodies regulate the use of the insulin.

The other piece of the consistency equation is the servings given from the food groups. If your child gets one protein and one carbohydrate every day for the morning snack don't deviate from that. But what you can do is provide many choices for the protein and carbohydrate and try different combinations.

If your child has a favourite meal or snack that works well with their blood sugar make it for them as often as they like. But they are going to get bored if they have to eat the same thing day in and day out. You are going to find that the food choices available are not as limited as you might have originally thought. You can also get creative and revamp old recipes making them friendly for diabetics by using sugar substitutes in place of sugar or using whole wheat in place of white (for instance in a pizza crust).

Browse diabetic cookbooks with your child and involve them in the meal planning. You are sure to have more success in preparing meals if they have a say in what they are eating.

Help From Grandparents With Diabetic Children

A night out on the town is just what mom and dad needs, but who is going to baby sit? Grandparents are the best baby sitters, especially when they involve an overnight stay. For parents of children with juvenile diabetes it might not be as easy. It is going to be hard to leave your child with anyone for an extended period of time unless they know how to take of your child and manage their diabetes.

Training and a little bit of practice is all that is needed. The good thing about grandparents is that you know they have your child's best interests at heart. They are going to take the responsibility seriously and follow your instructions to the letter.

To give the grandparents confidence and make yourself feel better do a trial run. Have a day where you are around and let grandma or grandpa take the reins for the day. It doesn't take much time to become comfortable with drawing and injecting the insulin and testing blood sugar levels with a monitor.

For the first visit, help out by providing a list of step-by-step instructions as a back-up. And you can even provide meal suggestions. Send your child with their emergency kit (they really shouldn't go anywhere without one anyway) and make sure everyone knows how and when to use the contents.

Leave contact numbers where you can be reached at all times. It will give peace of mind to everyone involved to know that if any questions arise or an emergency does develop you are just a phone call away. Encourage the calls so that no one feels that they are interrupting you – even for little questions.

After the first successful overnight stay, be ready for many more requests to go and stay at grandma and grandpa's house for a sleepover.

Of course, if one or the other grandparent is also diabetic, well, that would be a plus!

Insulin Pumps For Juvenile Diabetics

A popular alternative, especially for teenagers, to daily insulin injections is to use an insulin pump. Although it is an alternative for everyone because of the high cost of the unit and having to wear it 24 hours per day for others it can help in successfully managing juvenile diabetes.

An insulin pump is worn all the time and provides a steady stream of fast-acting insulin instead of a combination of fast-acting and long-lasting insulin that is typically combined in a syringe. If your child is has to have multiple needles in a day this is also an attractive alternative.

Wearing an insulin pump provides greater flexibility; there is no specific injection and eating times that have to be met. But eating at similar times each day is still recommended. One of the best features of wearing an insulin pump is the ability to bolus – giving additional fast-acting insulin immediately before eating a meal or a snack by pressing one of the buttons on the pump. This method can prevent spikes in blood sugar by providing a boost of insulin when it is needed most.

Some of the downsides of a pump are the expense. The unit itself is not cheap and you have to still buy the insulin and supplies to go with it. And it has to be worn all the time with the exception of bathing or swimming. But you and your child will have to weigh the pros and cons of a pump and see what they want to have in the end.

The same amount of effort is still needed to keep blood sugars in control but having an insulin pump can be more convenient by not having to worry about insulin injections. An insulin pump will also keep a steady stream of insulin in the body overnight when blood sugars can sometimes spike.

Juvenile Diabetes And Teenagers

Teenagers are young adults and are ready to take on new responsibilities. If your teenager has had juvenile diabetes for some time, this is the time to pass the reins of management over to them. It may seem a bit intimidating to you to let your child take control of their diabetes but it is the best thing you can do for them. They are approaching a time in their life when they are going to be going out on their own. For both your sake and theirs, a comfort level needs to be reached in reading blood sugars, giving injections and planning appropriate meals.

If your child was a teenager when he or she was first diagnosed, involve them in the process from the beginning. Their input and the ability to make some decisions will help them feel in control of a situation they would rather not be in.

The biggest point to stress and make sure your teenager understands is how important it is to keep proper control of their diabetes. Juvenile diabetes is a serious disease and it has serious complications if blood sugar levels are not kept under control.

Discuss with your child different scenarios that are sure to arise and try and come up with solutions or ways to manage them. Drinking can have a negative effect on blood glucose levels and it is important that a young adult realize the dangers. When they reach legal age, they need to know how drinking can affect them and ways to incorporate that into their life if they so choose.

As a parenting, letting go is a hard thing to do but it is necessary to create independent adults. Trust your child to make the right decisions for their diabetes and be there to guide them when necessary.

Treatment For Juvenile Diabetes

A child who is diagnosed with juvenile diabetes is going to need to follow a treatment plan for the rest of their life. But they will have a lot of support. And there have been many advances and improvements in the diabetic treatment industry in way of needles and monitoring devices.

Knowing your child's blood sugar level is crucial to good control of the disease. By using a monitor at home you will see if the diet and insulin that is being provided is sufficient. There are many brands of monitors available and the amount of blood required is a very small drop placed on a strip. The monitor will come with a lancet device to draw the blood from a fingertip – it is relatively painless and takes very little time.

In order to replace or supplement the insulin in your child's body, a daily injection (sometimes more) is going to be required. In some cases a child will need more than one needle if the insulin from one is not lasting the entire day. You will learn how to monitor and adjust the level of insulin your child receives based on their blood glucose levels and advice from your doctor.

The other part of treating diabetes in children is a balanced diet and plenty of physical activity. Follow the food guide for children and limit the amount of treats that they are given. Daily exercise will help children maintain a healthy weight which in turns helps to control their blood sugar by limiting the amount of insulin they need. After a little bit of time treating diabetes will become a way of life for you and your child. Expect an adjustment period in the beginning but it will get better as you learn more and get the diabetes under control.

Juvenile Diabetes In Younger Children

When younger children are diagnosed with juvenile diabetes is can be very hard on them. They may not understand the severity of the disease and all of the restrictions that are placed on them. It is going to take patience and time for them to get used to their new lifestyle and the changes that go with it. Here are some tips to make the transition a little easier.

Join a support group of other parents whose children have been diagnosed with juvenile diabetes. Their experience in dealing with situations that you are going through can help to give your ideas and let you know that you are not alone on this journey. Not only can this type of group benefit the parents, it is for the children too. It will be beneficial for them to have friends that have diabetes too. As they grow older, these friendships can last a lifetime based on the common link of juvenile diabetes.

In the beginning especially you may feel guilt because you are constantly saying no to your child. It is for their own good that they can't have treats whenever they want but it doesn't make it any easier. Steel yourself against the cries, begging, and whining that may ensue and know that it will get easier as time goes on. Change is difficult for many including kids.

As your child get older and has more experience under their belt, involve them in the process of managing their diabetes. This will help them feel more in control of their disease and as the same time prepare them for the time when they are going to be on their own and have to take care of their own injections and blood glucose monitoring.

Each child is different and is going to handle the changes in their own way. Be there to support and help your child in whatever way they need.

The Risk Factors For Juvenile Diabetes

Although there is no known cause for juvenile diabetes there are risk factors that can contribute to the likeliness a child will be diagnosed with the disease. As some forms of type 1 diabetes are an autoimmune disease you can be at a higher risk if you have already been diagnosed with a different autoimmune disease. There are also some conditions surrounding a mother's pregnancy and labour than could contribute to the diagnosis of juvenile diabetes.

If your child has been diagnosed with one of these autoimmune disease he or she is considered at a higher risk for diabetes in childhood:

* If your child has had one of these viruses: hepatitis, mumps, or CMV disease * Thyroid problems known as hypothyroidism or hyperthyroidism (or Graves' disease) * Celiac disease

There has been some evidence that has shown that a child born to a mother over the age of 35 could be at higher risk for developing type 1 diabetes. This is not conclusive and it is not to say that a child born to a younger mother is not at risk as well. Some studies indicate that a mother who had pre-eclampsia during pregnancy will give birth to a baby with a higher risk of being diagnosed – but this is not a proven fact.

Other risk factors include race - people from Northern Europe or areas of the Mediterranean – are considered at higher risk than other races. Environmental and dietary factors can play a role too. If a child is under a lot of stress it is considered a reason why he or she may go onto develop type 1 diabetes. Dietary risks factors include high levels of dairy and nitrosamines (used as a preservative in some meats and cheeses). Exposure to toxins is considered a risk factor too.

What Do To When A Child With Juvenile Diabetes Gets Sick

It's never fun when a child gets sick with a cold or flu. They don't feel good, sometimes get grumpy and need to be taken care of. This is true for a child with juvenile diabetes too, but there is the added concern of how their blood glucose levels will be affected by the illness. This is just another hurdle to deal with once your child has been diagnosed with diabetes.

If you are giving your child an over-the-counter or prescription medicine be sure to read the labels and warning or talk to the pharmacist. Some medications will cause a child's blood sugar to be elevated and this should be taken into account when planning insulin dosage and meal plans.

If your child is sick and has no appetite or is vomiting, it is still important that they take their insulin. By testing their blood sugar frequently you can determine an adjusted amount of insulin to give them but don't skip it entirely. If your child's blood sugar is too low and they cannot eat anything try giving them a soda that is not sugar free.

Keep in mind that when your child is ill or stressed (or both) their blood sugar will be raised by that alone. If you are unsure how to help your child or you cannot get their blood sugars under control, call your doctor for advice.

When your child is sick, check their ketones more often than just in the morning when they have fasted. If they are not eating because of nausea they could be spilling ketones into their urine and suffer from ketoacidosis. This is a serious condition that needs medical attention. Make sure your child is receiving their regular insulin injections and are drinking plenty of fluids in order to prevent this condition from developing.

Traveling And Juvenile Diabetes

Planning on a family vacation? Don't worry trips and other family outings do not have to be restricted because your child has been diagnosed with juvenile diabetes. You can do it all still but there are some extra preparations and planning that will have to happen first. The preparations you make is going to be dependent on what kind of trip you are planning, for how long and the activities that you will be participating in.

It is a good idea if you are going out of town on an airplane or by car to get some documentation from your doctor. You should get a letter that explains your child's condition and an extra prescription for any unforeseen eventualities. If you are going on a lengthy plane ride, you will need the letter to get permission to bring your child's medicine and syringes onto the airplane with you instead of storing them in your luggage.

If you are unsure what special arrangements you are going to need to make, speak to your doctor. If you are going on a vacation that will involve lots of extra physical activity (such as camping or hiking), be sure that you bring extra food to replace the energy that is going to be used up. If there is going to be less physical activity, more frequent testing of blood sugar levels will be necessary to make sure too much insulin isn't being used.

When traveling a distance that involves crossing different time zones, be prepared to make additional adjustments to your child's eating schedule. No matter what the clock says, your child is going to need their insulin and food on their body's time. Again, your doctor can help you make a plan for this adjustment and it will be based on the length of your trip, the difference in time zones, and your child.

Products For Diabetic Children

Diabetes strikes at any age. But one type of diabetes is particularly notorious towards very young patients. It's called juvenile diabetes. Although juvenile diabetes is not exclusive among children, it's relatively high prevalence in the younger population make it a root of concern for parents whose children were diagnosed with this chronic, insulin-dependent condition. There are many things that a child with juvenile diabetes needs. Some of them are discussed below:

Blood glucose meter or glucometer – The first and one that should be at the top of your list of priorities is the glucometer. This is a portable device that measures the glucose levels in the blood of the patient. You don't normally have to pay a high price to get this device since manufacturers sell these at a very low price. Also, many insurance companies provide coverage for this device. When considering a particular brand or model, it is best to first check the price and availability of compatible test strips. This is because these strips usually have a huge cut on the expenses incurred on monitoring blood glucose levels. Test strips are usually priced at $1 per piece, but it is not uncommon to find 50 cent per piece strips.

Insulin pen – An insulin pen is a portable insulin delivery system that looks very much like a regular pen. This injects controlled doses of insulin into the bloodstream without the need for a health care personnel's assistance. There are two types of insulin pens: the pre-filled pen and the durable pen. The former is a disposable pen that contains pre-mixed insulin and the latter is a pen that only needs cartridge replacements. There is, however, a new type of insulin pen that has built-in memory. This can contain up to a hundred values which should make recording of time, date and insulin dosage easier for the user.

Emergency glucose tablet – This diabetic product for children is one way of controlling insulin reaction. Whereas adults use candy and other sweets, diabetic children are administered with emergency glucose tablets that deliver precise amounts of glucose into the bloodstream to normalize blood glucose levels. Although a lot of people see these as candy substitutes, these do not look candy at all so parents and teachers will not have any problem with missing glucose tablets.

Insulin pump – Otherwise known as continuous subcutaneous insulin infusion therapy, an insulin pump is a medical device that is used to administer insulin to treat symptoms of diabetes mellitus. This device comprises of a pump, a disposable reservoir that is attached inside the pump, and a disposable infusion set. Taking the price out of the equation, an insulin pump is a good alternative to daily injections of insulin using injections products since it makes a person do away with multiple insulin injections. When used alongside a carb counting device and a blood glucose monitoring device, this can make for an intensive insulin therapy.

Injection products – Many children run away from injection products like syringes and needles. This should not be the case, however. Parents should help condition their children's thinking towards injection products.

Lancets and lancet devices – These are devices used to draw blood samples for blood glucose testing. The priority in choosing these products is to find those that could give the least discomfort to their users.

Juvenile Diabetes And The Honeymoon Period

In many children with juvenile diabetes a period occurs shortly after being diagnosed they go through what is commonly called as the honeymoon period. This is a time when your child's blood sugar levels will return to normal without the aid of additional insulin. It is important to remember that this happens in a lot of children and does not mean that the disease has gone away. The pancreas is still trying to do its job and is working overtime to make insulin for your child's body. Following are some guidelines to follow when this happens.

The length of the honeymoon period is not the same for everyone. In one child it can last months while in another child it can feasibly last for over a year. It all depends on how much insulin your child's pancreas can produce and how long it can keep up that rate of production. It will be hard to figure out how much if any insulin your child needs during this time when their blood sugar levels are normal. Constant monitoring of the blood glucose levels is still required, because you will not know when the honeymoon period is over otherwise.

Keep in close contact with your health care provider. He or she will help in determining what the best plan is to follow during the honeymoon phase. Some may even want you to give minute amounts of insulin daily in order to keep your child used to the injections and your child's body accustomed to the additional insulin it will need.

It can be emotionally hard for your child during the honeymoon phase. Everything will seem back to normal and they are going to want to resume their life like it was prior to diagnosis. It is important to remain on the diabetic diet and continue monitoring during this time.

When Choosing A Blood Glucose Meter For Children

Blood glucose meter is a portable device is something that all diabetics cannot live without. Constantly monitoring blood glucose fluctuations is very important since blood glucose values often dictate how the healthcare team attending the patient can best deliver treatment.

But, blood glucose monitoring is most important for parents whose children were diagnosed with diabetes, specifically type 1 diabetes or insulin-dependent diabetes. These parents need to monitor their children's glucose levels so that appropriate measures can be set in place and so that the onset of symptoms can be staved off. But, above all, children who depend entirely on insulin injections need to keep watch of their blood glucose levels. Doing so will not only help them find a rest from constantly shooting up blood glucose levels, but will help them function more normally.

So what is type 1 diabetes? Also called juvenile diabetes, type 1 diabetes is a condition that is characterized by the pancreas' lack of capacity to produce its own insulin. Insulin is the hormone that allows the delivery of glucose into individual cells to give them energy. Without this ability, all cells in the body will lack the energy to continue performing at their optimal capacity, leaving the patient very weak and bodily functions compromised. Also, without insulin, the bloodstream will be flooded with so much glucose or sugar, which leads to a host of uncomfortable diabetes symptoms.

To prevent symptoms like frequent urination, increased thirst, increased appetite, constant fatigue and others, patients to keep blood glucose levels under control. Among the best ways of doing so is by using blood glucose meter.

Blood glucose meter comes in all shapes and sizes, and depending on the manufacturer and brand, in a variety of technologies. To know which one can help the patient best, the following pointers can be considered:

Cost

This device come in cheap, in fact, many manufacturers even give it away for free. So you shouldn't be paying a lot for a blood glucose meter. But, remember that these companies do not give their products away at a very low cost because of purely altruistic reasons. You should beware of the test strips that are used alongside this device. When considering a blood glucose meter, check first the price of the test strips that are compatible with the product. This should be anywhere from 50 cents to one dollar per strip. You might use three or more of these strips every day to continually monitor your child's blood glucose levels.

Insurance

Like blood glucose meters manufacturers, insurance companies also provide coverage for the device, but not usually on the test strips. Be sure to check with your provider regarding the coverage your kid will get in terms of his diabetic expenses.

Ease of use

Look for convenience when buying a glucometer. Your child should be able to use it on his own without supervision to see whether it is easy enough to be used. It should also be light enough to be carried around since your kid will have to take it with him on a constant basis. If you or your child has vision problems, it is best to stick with a glucometer that has a mid-sized to large display screen so both of you would not have difficulty reading the values.

Built-in memory

Some blood glucose meters come with built-in memory that is powerful enough to record up to a few hundred readings. If your kid manages to be with his own a lot, you should try getting him one that has good memory capacity so you can keep track of the trends on the fluctuations of blood glucose levels.

Celebrating Special Occasions And Juvenile Diabetes

You may be worried about the long-term effects on your child once they are diagnosed with diabetes but their immediate concerns may be quite different. It is natural for them to focus on things they can't have anymore or might miss out on. Such as cake and ice cream at birthday parties, candy from Halloween, and a big dinner with pie at Thanksgiving and Christmas. But being diabetic does not mean that you have to abstain from all sweets all the time.

Plan and plan some more. If you know that your child is going to be going to a birthday party on Saturday afternoon, alter their food intake for that day to allow them to have a small piece of cake. Until your children are much older, it is a good idea for you to stay with them at a birthday party in case of any emergencies.

If there is a class party at the school, volunteer to make something that the class can share and your child can have safely. If your children's teachers are aware of the special dietary requirements they can include sugar-free treats on special occasions.

The same holds true for Christmas and Thanksgiving as for birthday parties. Planning ahead and adjusting meals earlier in the day will allow your child to participate in all of the festivities at holiday time that revolve around food. There are many recipes and variations to recipes that are considered diabetic friendly. These include cakes, pies, and other desserts.

There are things that can be done so your child does not feel deprived. It will make the transition smoother for everyone if you can continue on with life with only while integrated the changes needed for someone living with diabetes. But the allowances should not be made every day – keep them to special occasions only.

ABOUT THE AUTHOR

Robert Rumball initially contracted Stress Diabetes when hospitalised in a Burns Ward for 3 months in 1980. This cleared up before he was discharged, but re-appeared several years later as Type 2 Diabetes, and he still lives with this today.

Robert had to regretfully, give up his gold prospecting a few years ago because of painful knee joints, so he settled down to write articles and books. This sedentary lifestyle soon had its price, Diabetic Peripheral Neuropathy, which affects both feet, his hands, and his torso.

Knowing absolutely nothing about Peripheral Neuropathy, he has spent countless hours researching it, as well as the various forms that Diabetes takes.

This book is the product of that research.

Robert also has published two websites that could interest you:
http://footpain-diabetic.com
http://herbal-remedies-for.com

www.ingramcontent.com/pod-product-compliance
Lightning Source LLC
Chambersburg PA
CBHW060223290526
45789CB00003B/1382